ISBN: 1979531269
ISBN-13: 978-1979531269

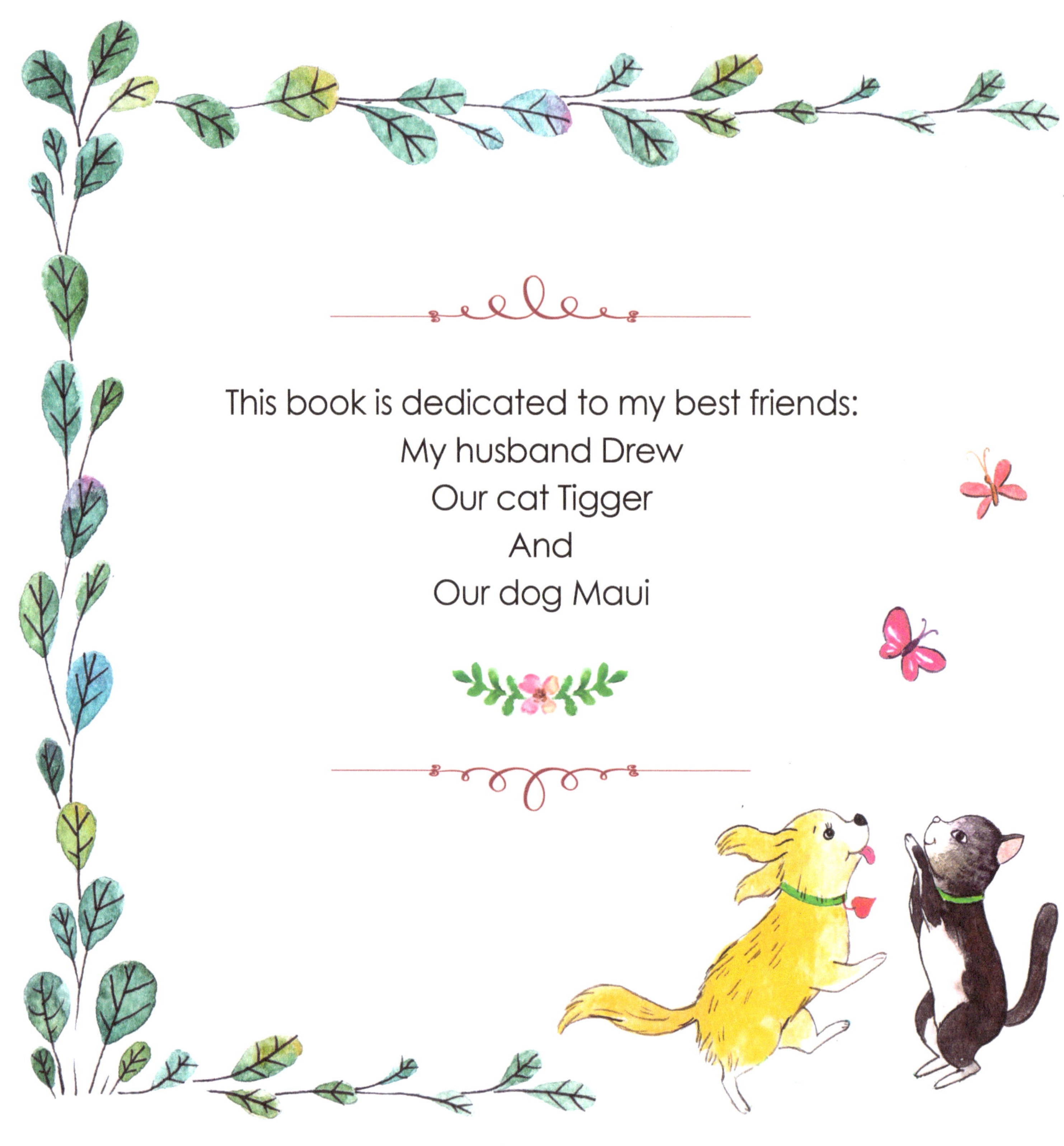

This book is dedicated to my best friends:
My husband Drew
Our cat Tigger
And
Our dog Maui

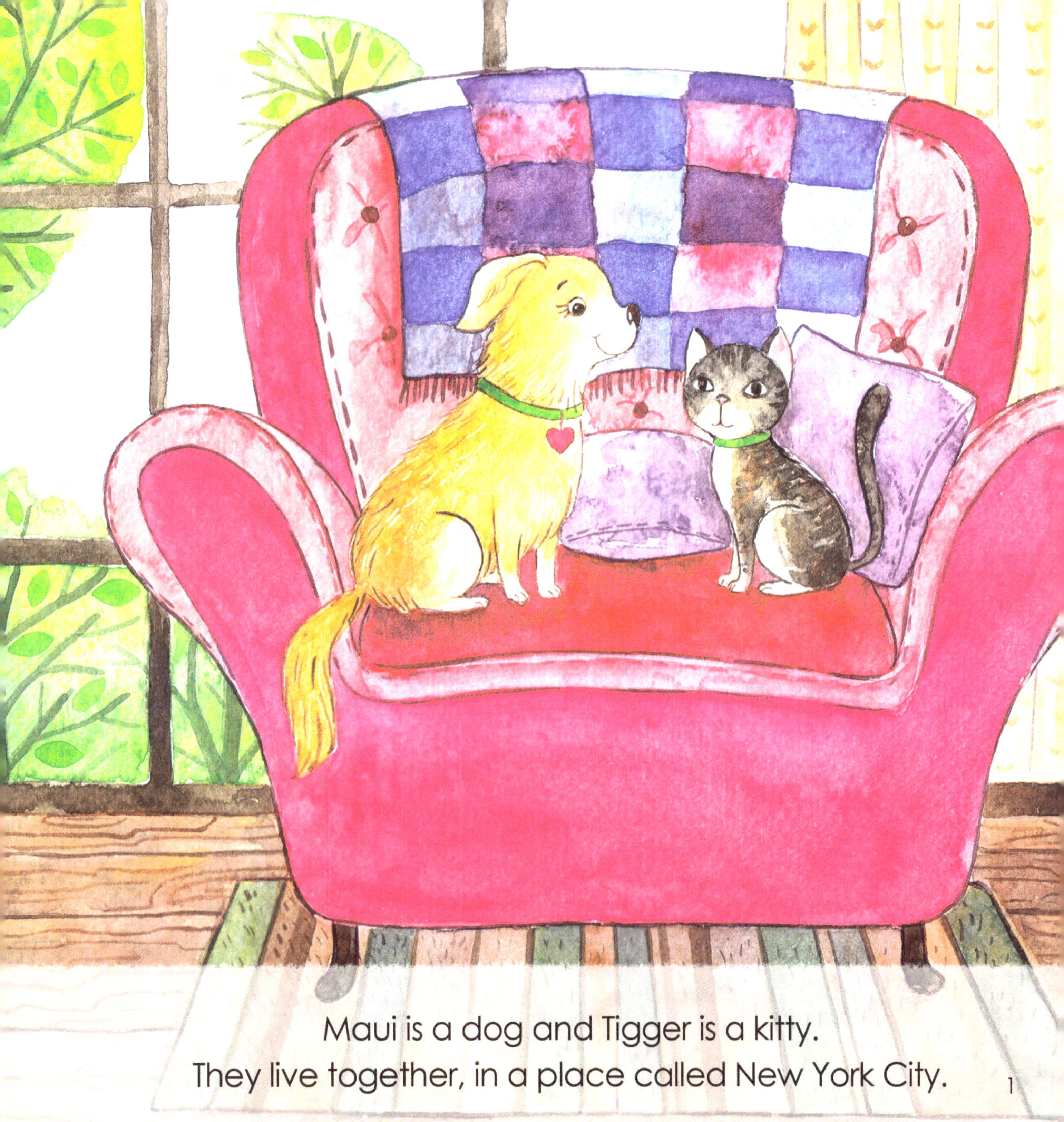

Maui is a dog and Tigger is a kitty.
They live together, in a place called New York City.

One day Maui and Tigger began to play. They started at home, but then lost their way.

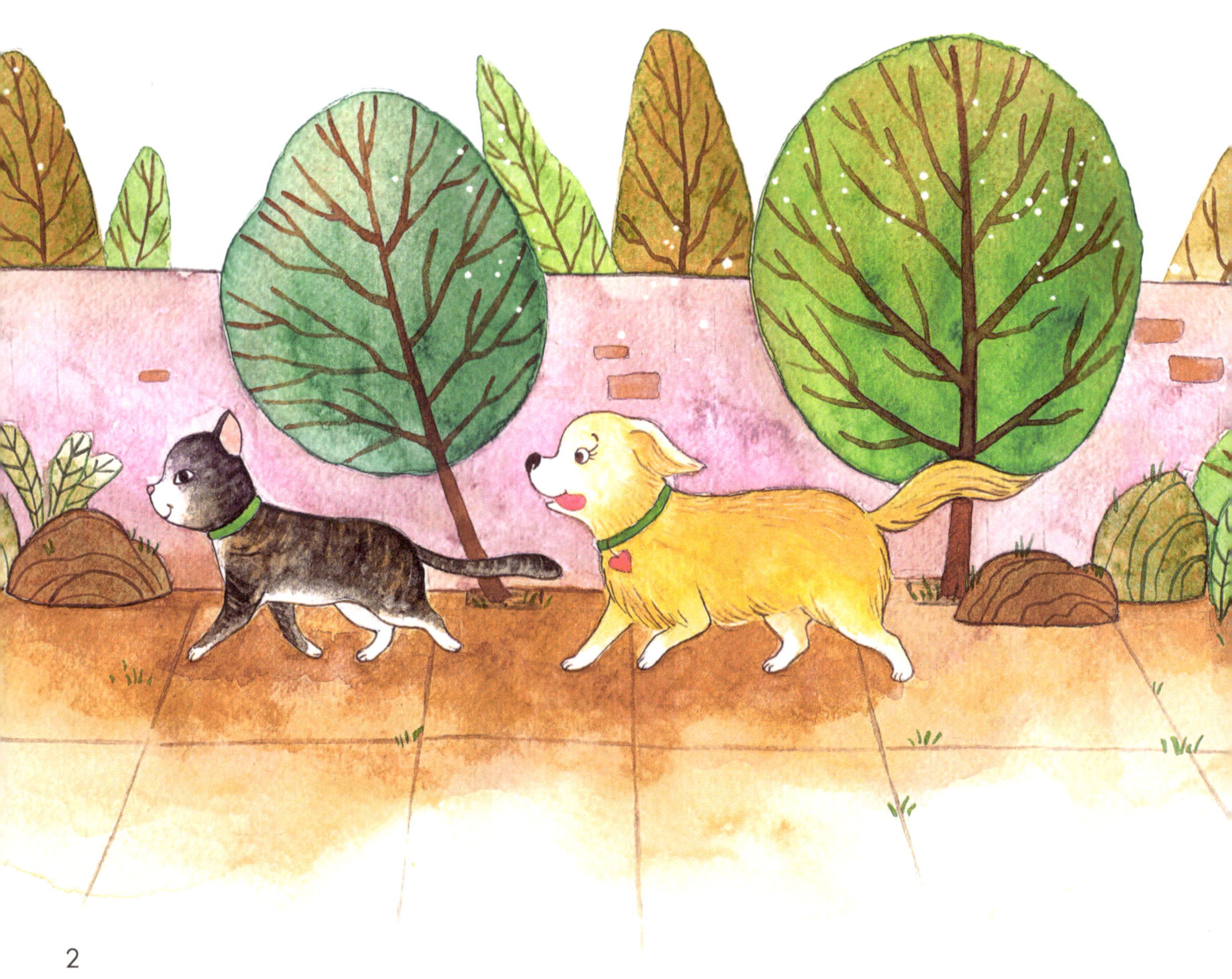

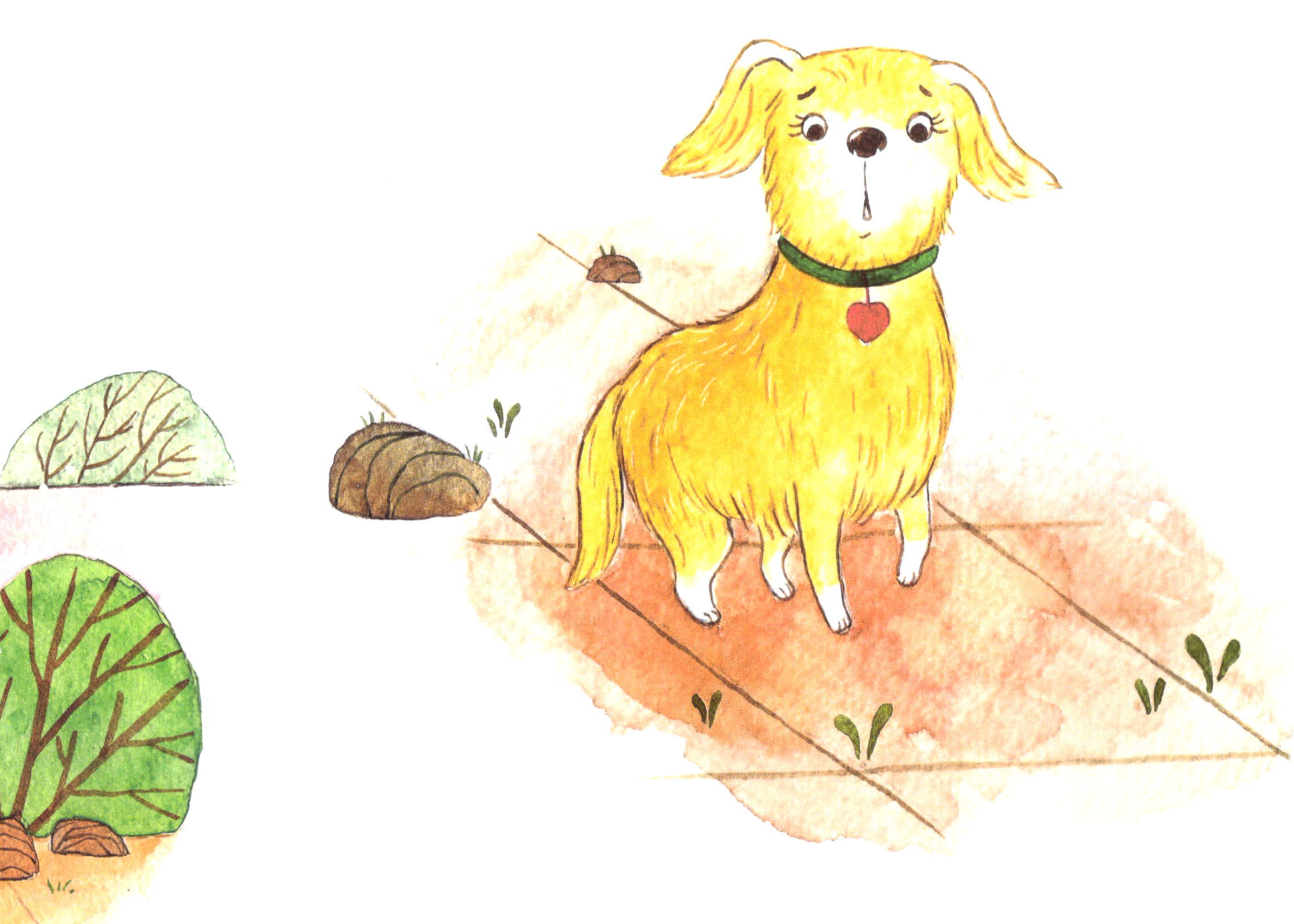

Maui looked up and shouted "OH NO!"
"Tigger, we're outside! Which way do we go?"

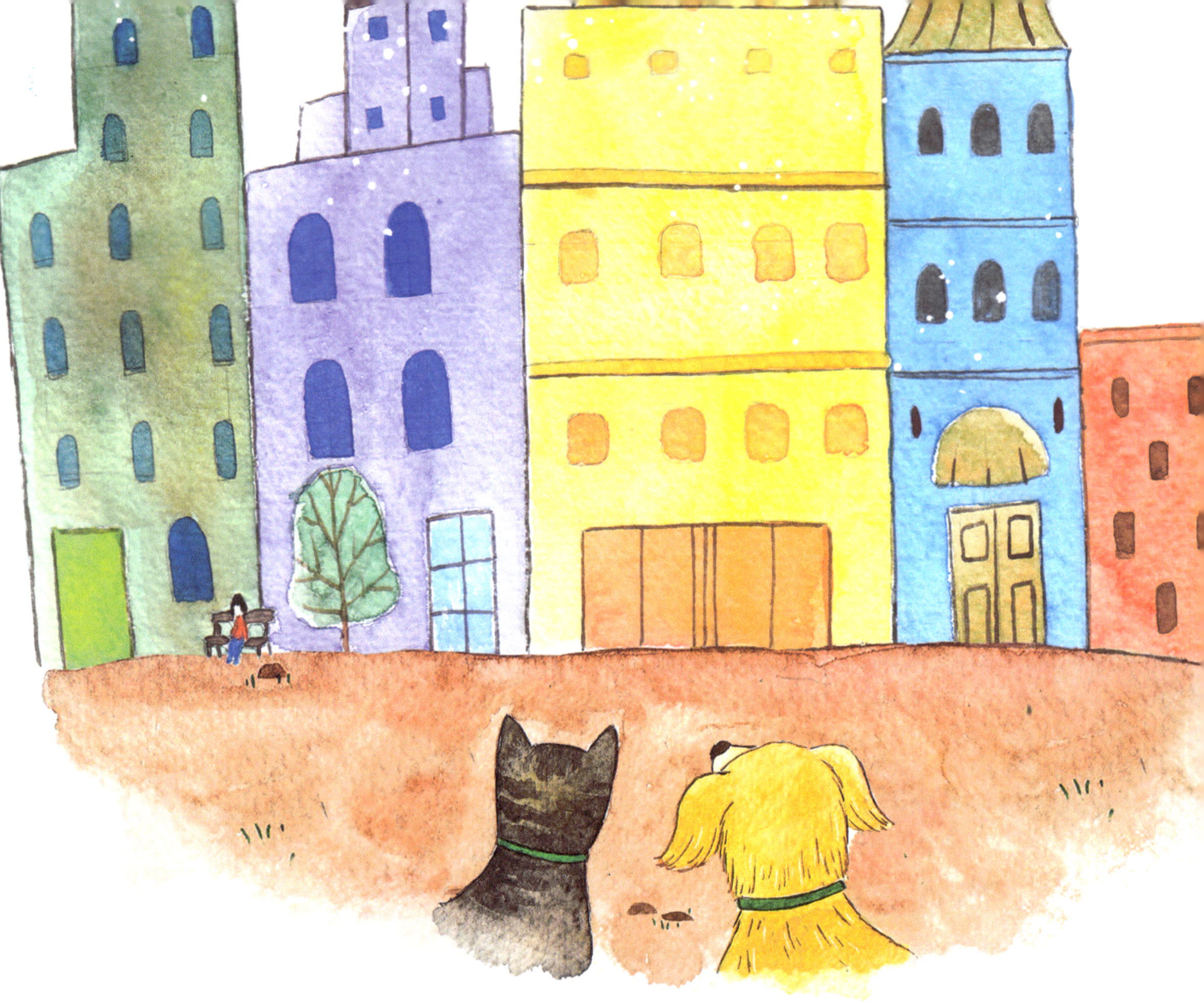

Tigger looked all around but all she could see were buildings, and people, and one little tree.

"I don't know," said Tigger, "But we must get back home."

"Or our parents will worry, and cry, and moan."

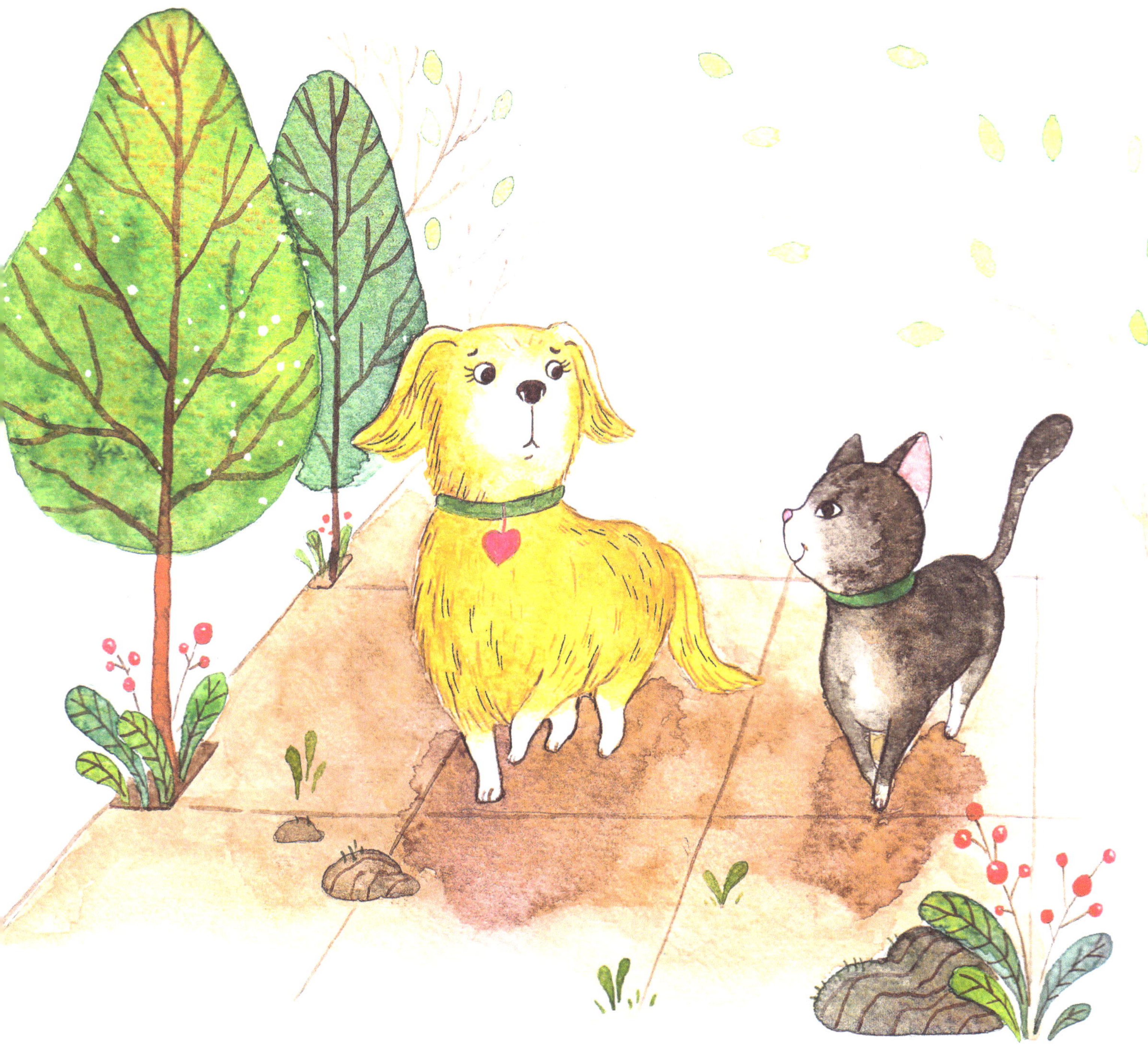

"I'm so scared!" exclaimed Maui, "But I don't know why."
"I'm feeling real dizzy and I think I might cry!"

"It's alright." said Tigger, "Things can sometimes be scary."
"But I have a game, that will help you be merry!"

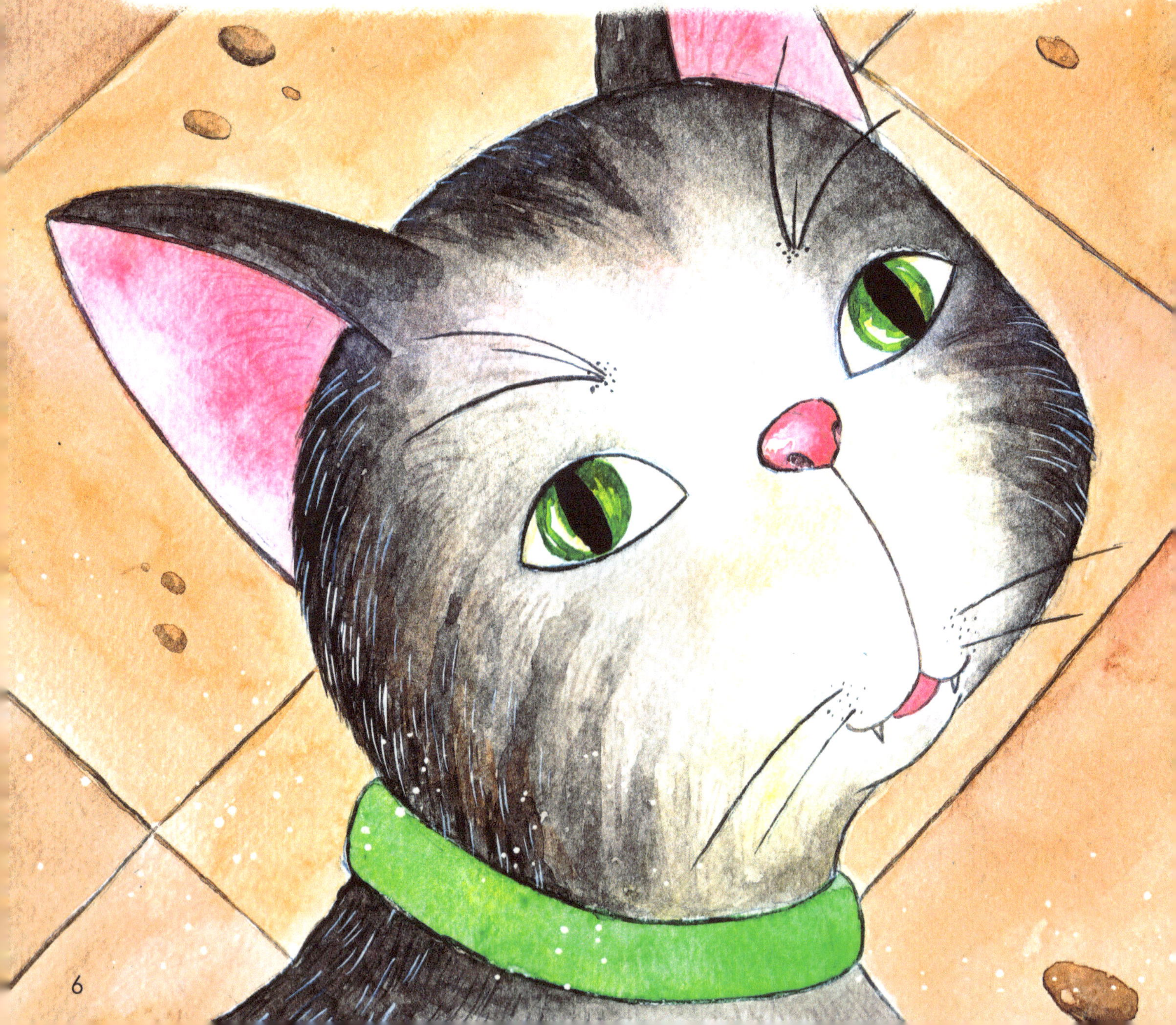

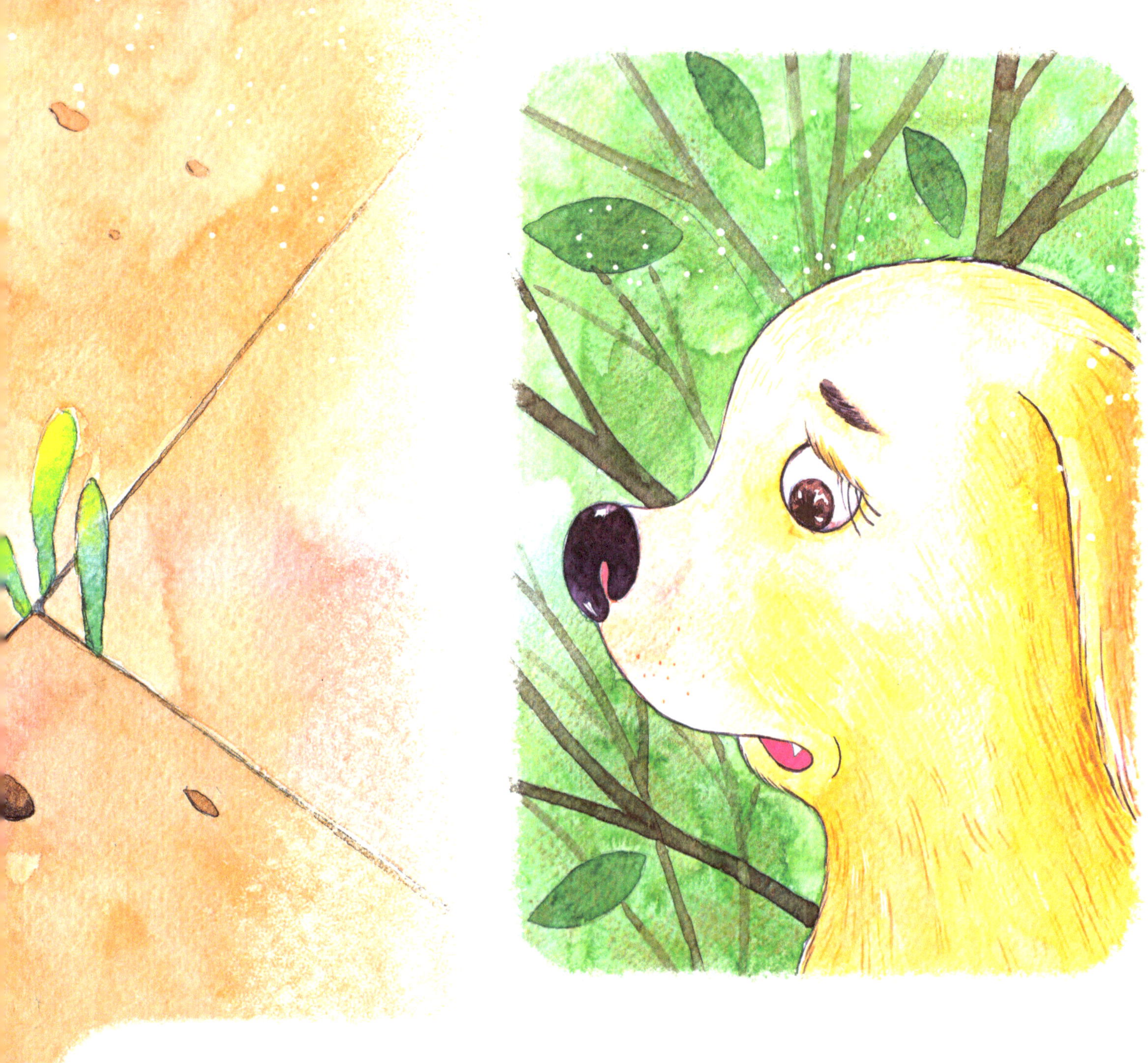

"A game?" asked Maui, "There's no time for this! We're lost! We're lost! And soon we'll be missed!"

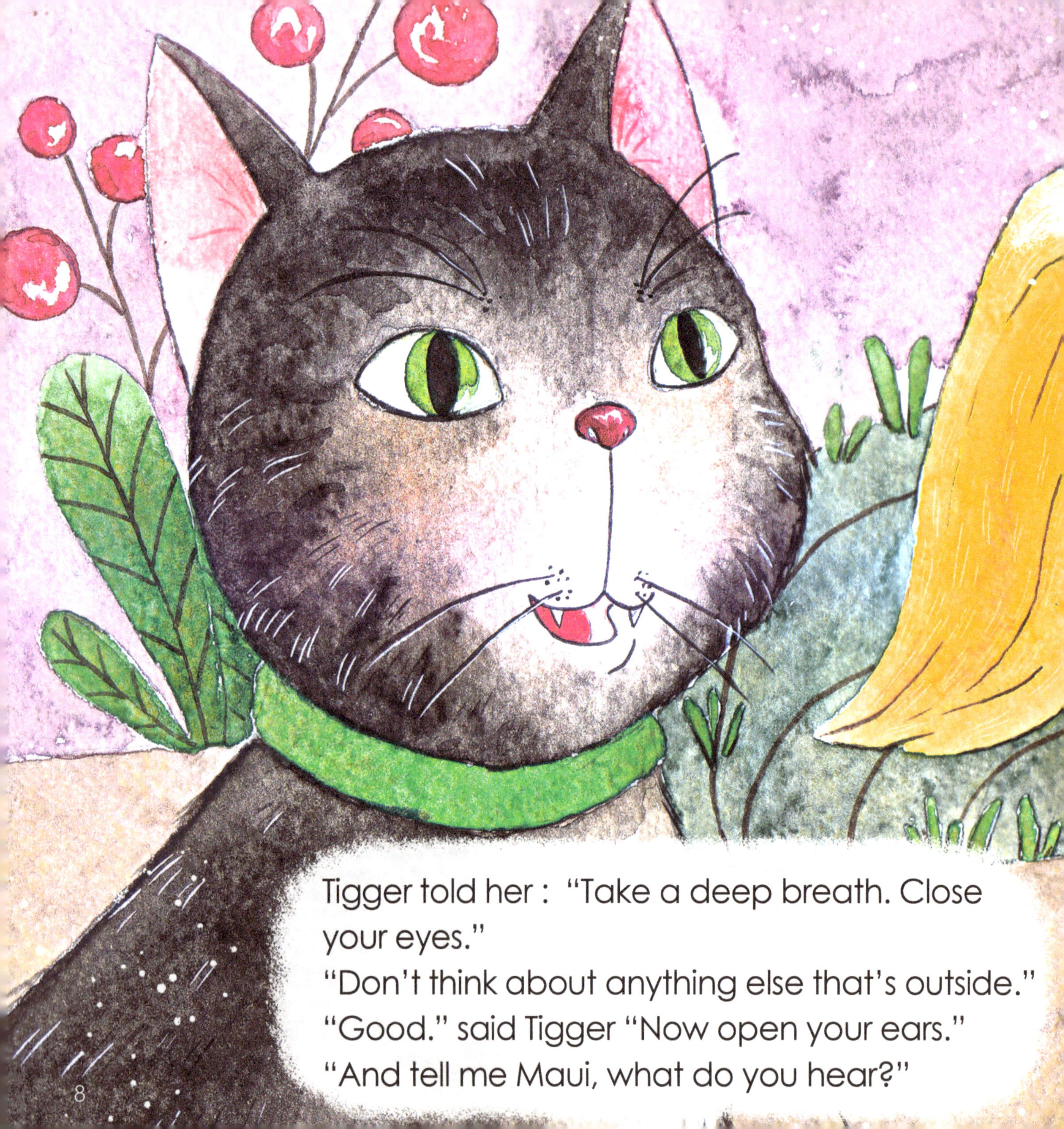

Tigger told her : "Take a deep breath. Close your eyes."
"Don't think about anything else that's outside."
"Good." said Tigger "Now open your ears."
"And tell me Maui, what do you hear?"

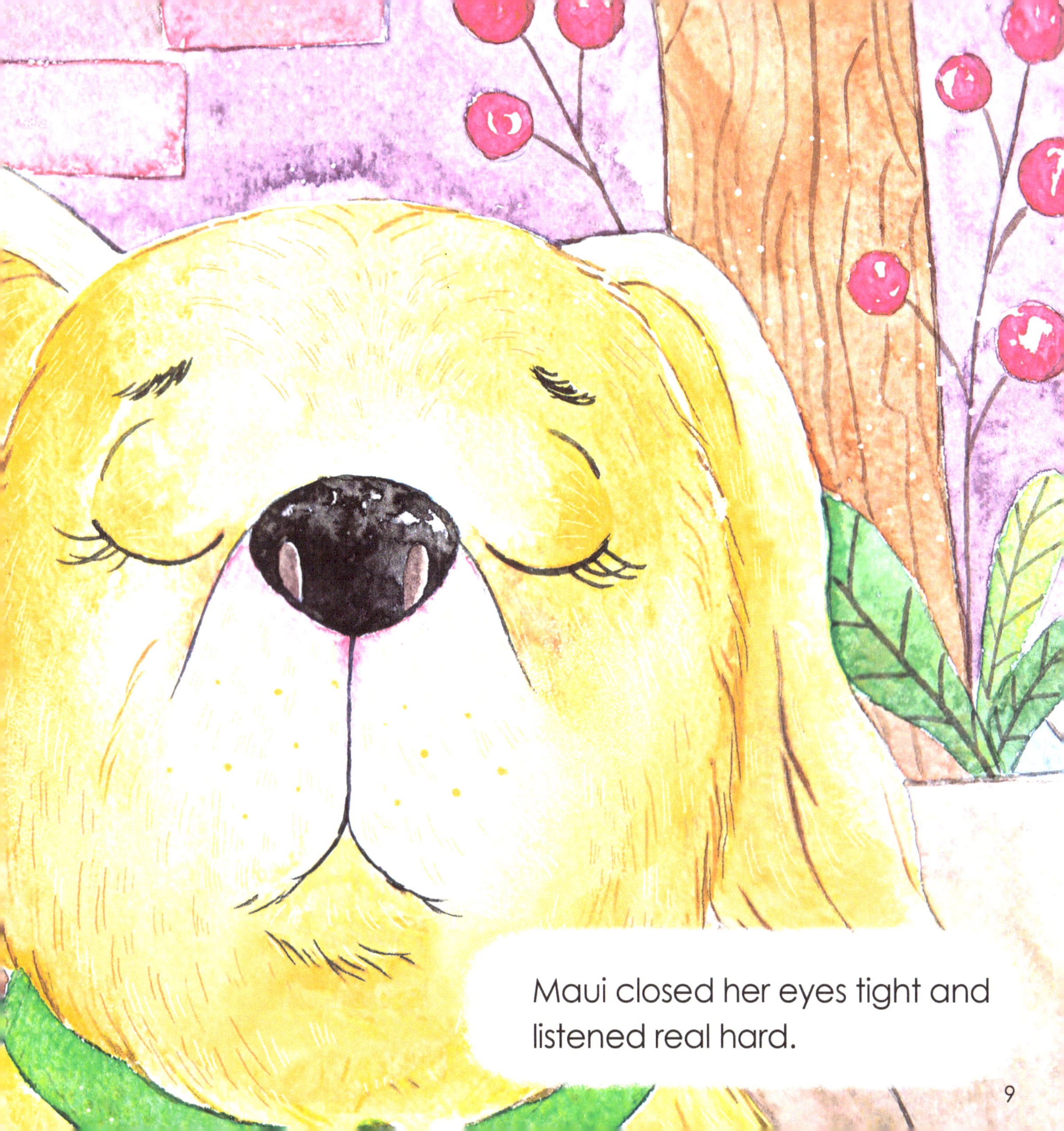

Maui closed her eyes tight and listened real hard.

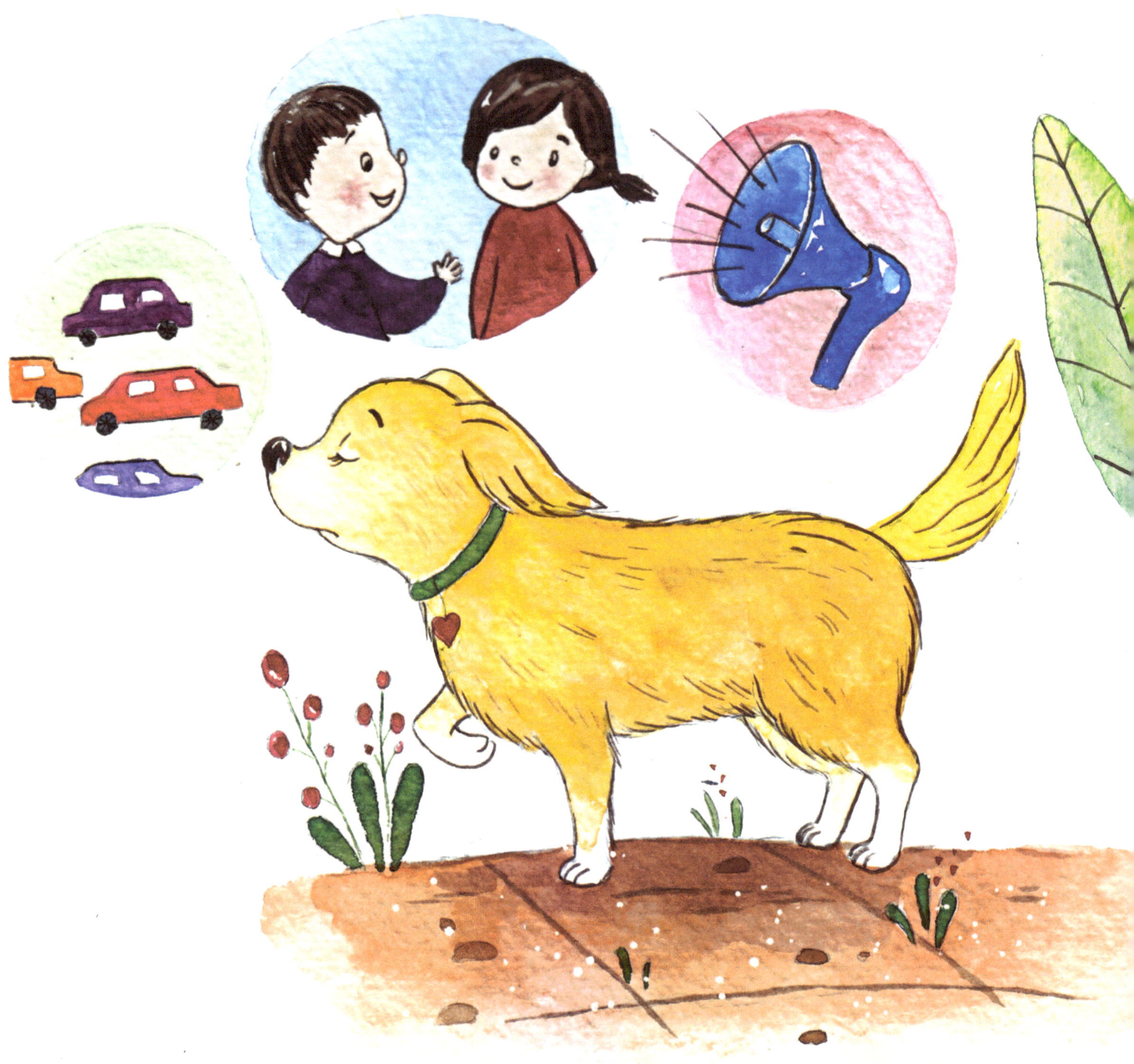

"I hear people, and sirens, and a whole bunch of cars."

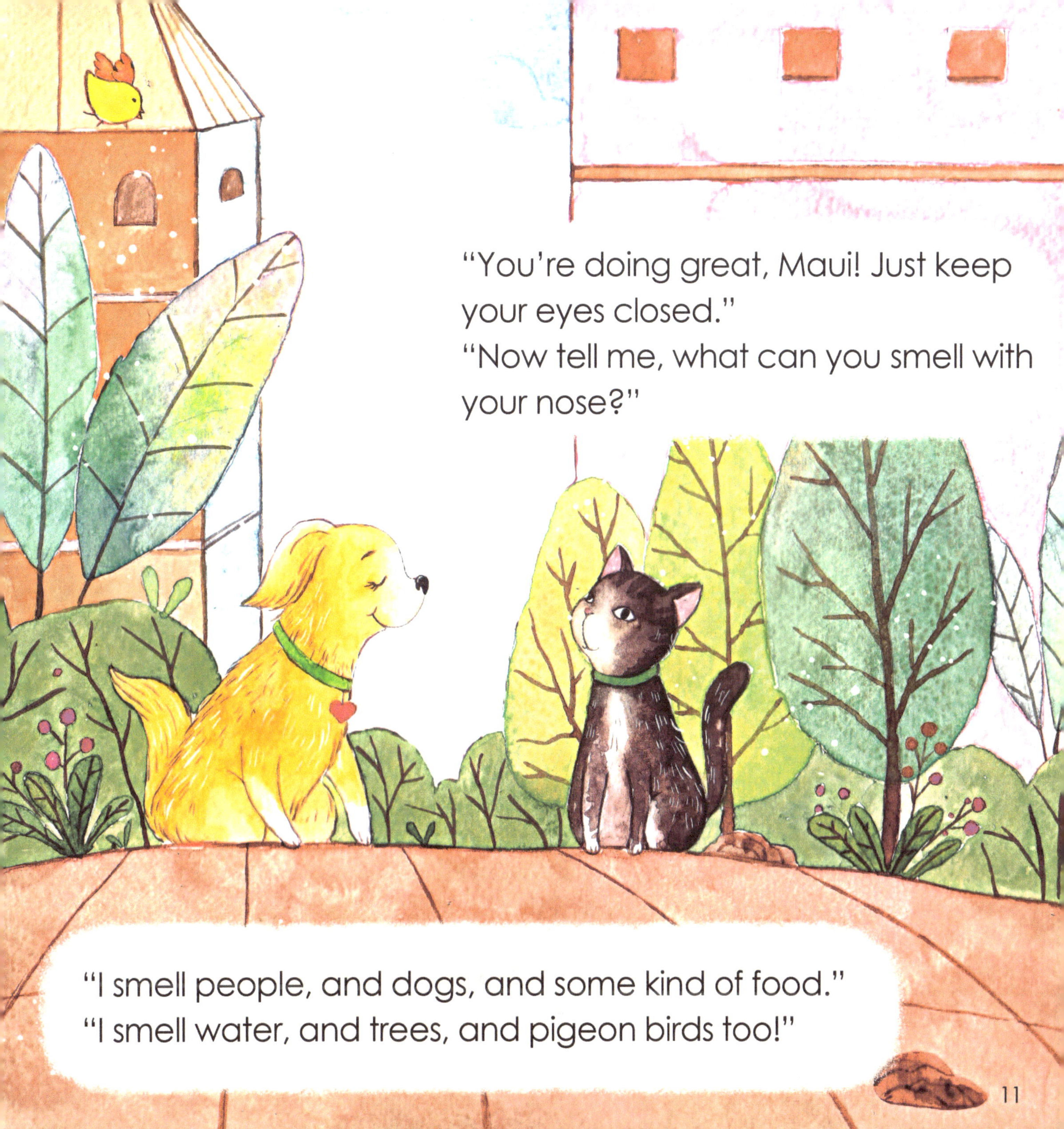

"You're doing great, Maui! Just keep your eyes closed."
"Now tell me, what can you smell with your nose?"
"I smell people, and dogs, and some kind of food."
"I smell water, and trees, and pigeon birds too!"

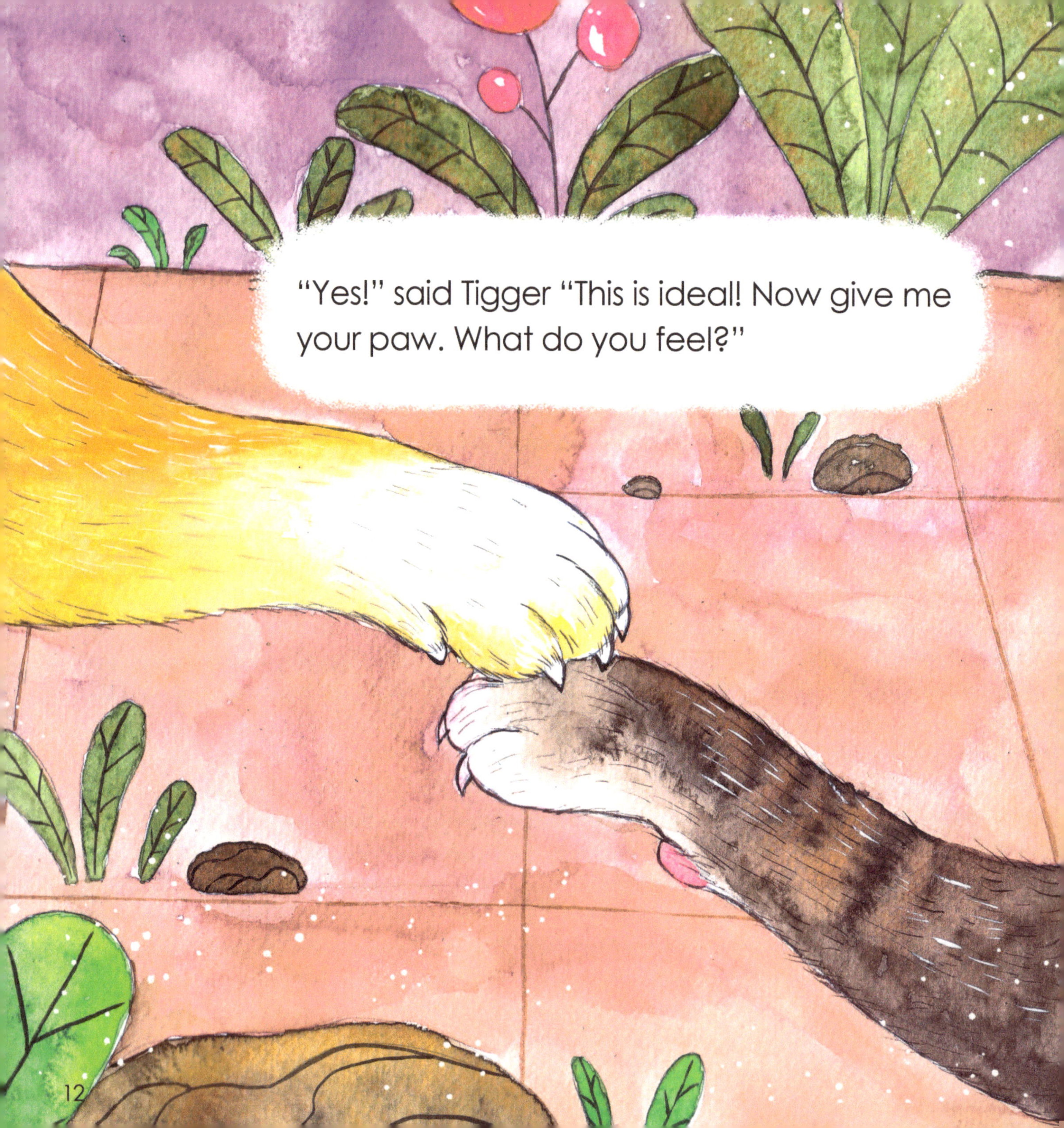

"Yes!" said Tigger "This is ideal! Now give me your paw. What do you feel?"

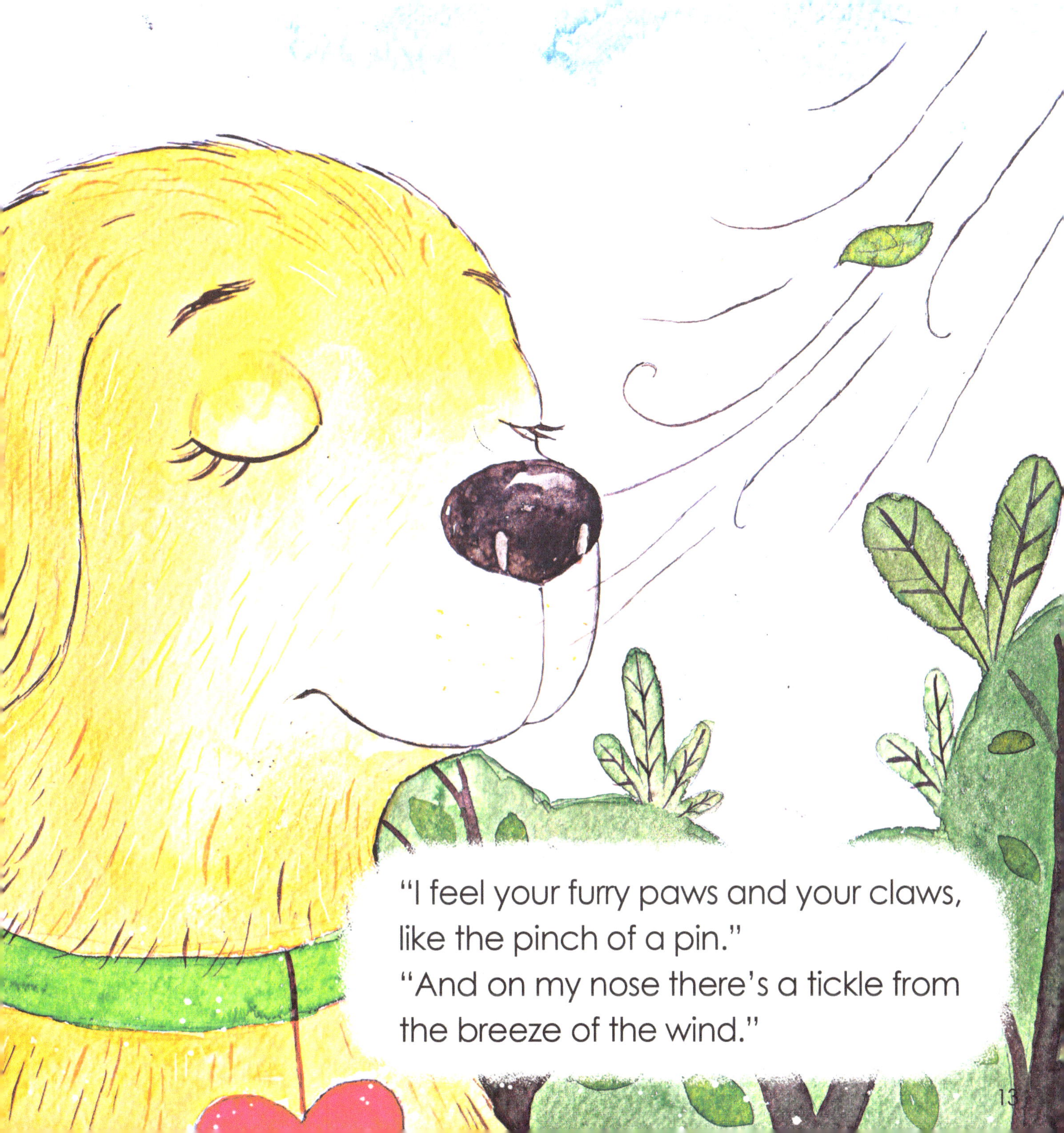

"I feel your furry paws and your claws,
like the pinch of a pin."
"And on my nose there's a tickle from
the breeze of the wind."

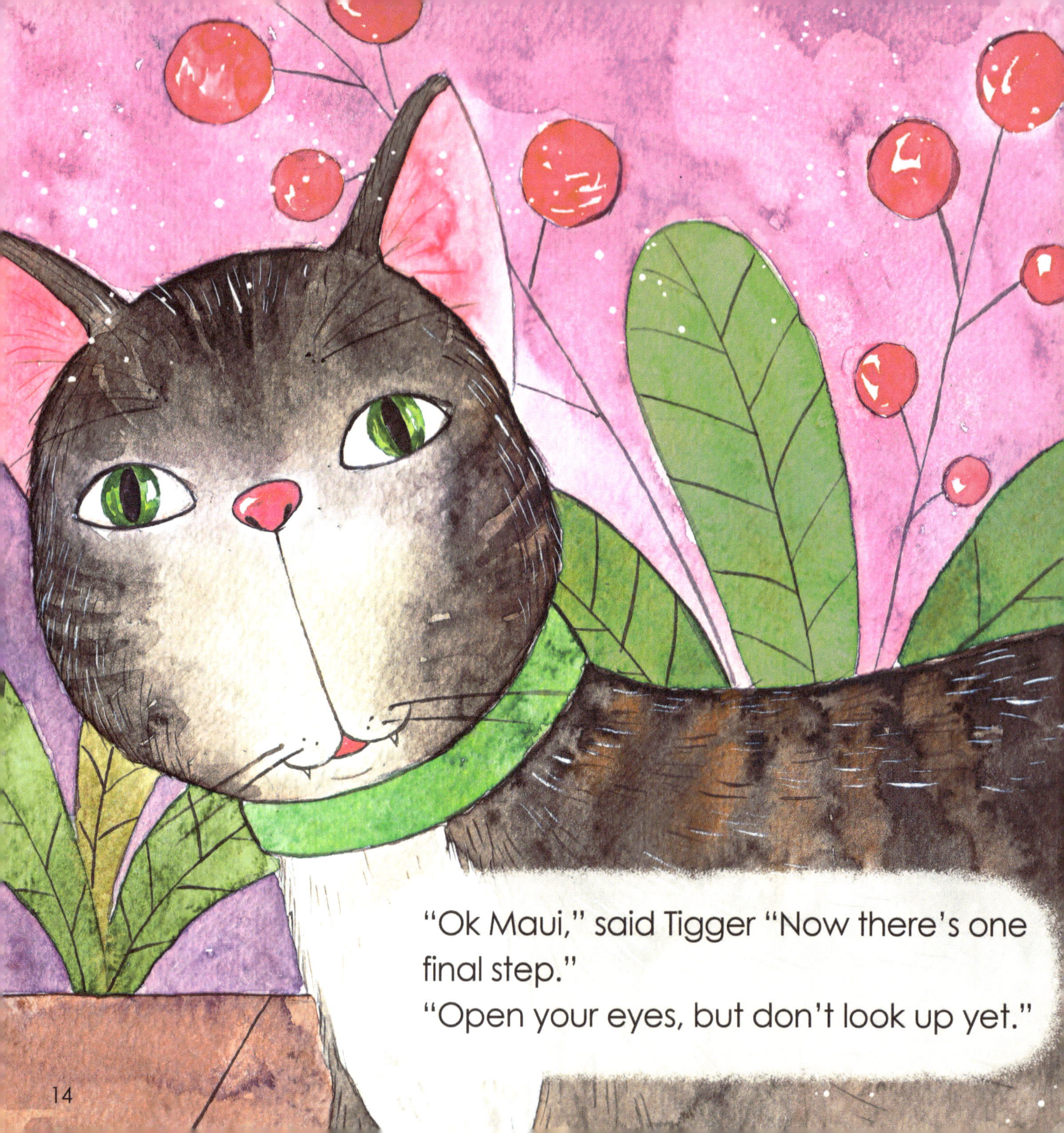
"Ok Maui," said Tigger "Now there's one final step."
"Open your eyes, but don't look up yet."

"Wow!" said Maui "This isn't so hard!"
"And I'm feeling much better than I did at the start."

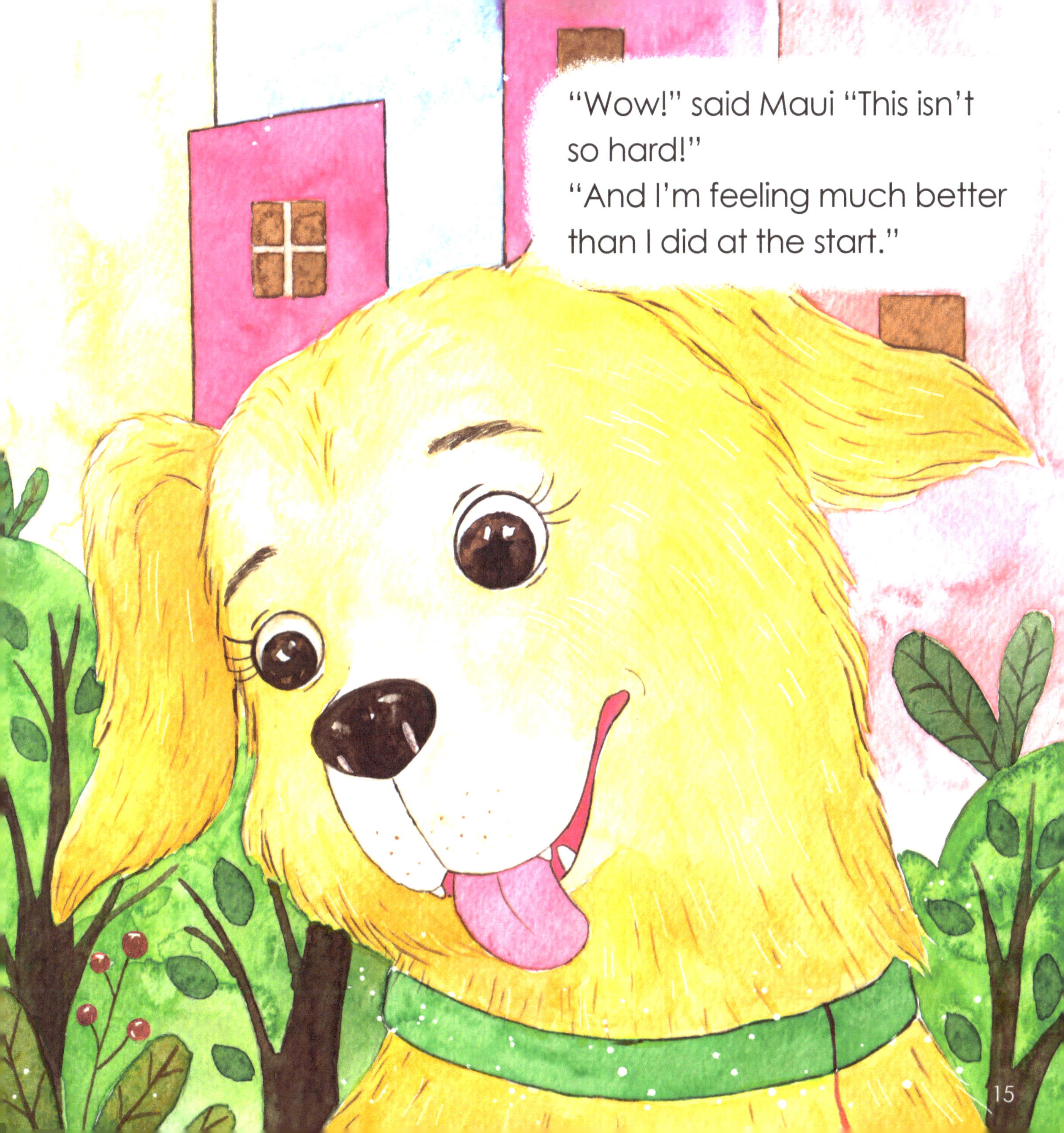

15

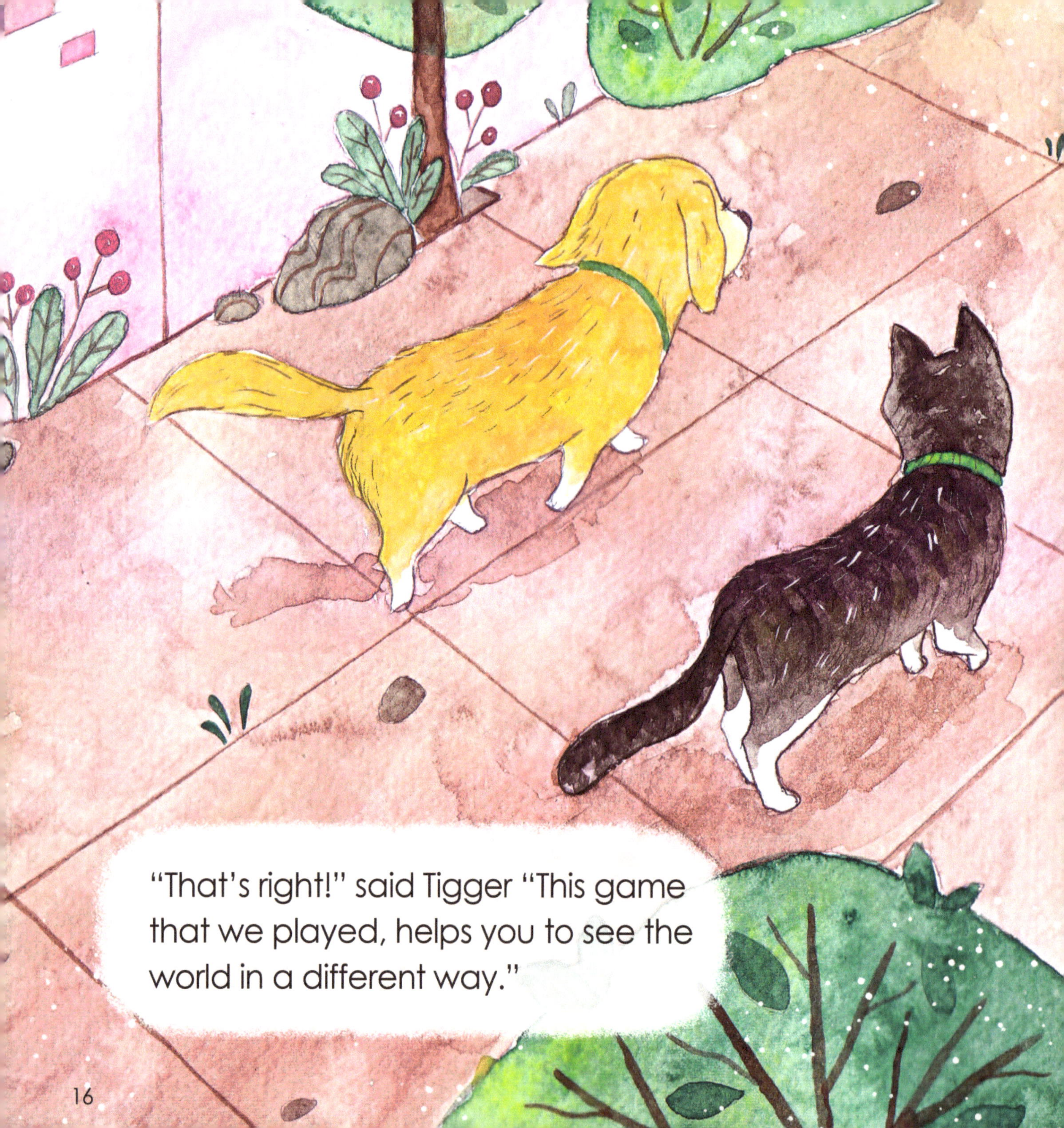

"That's right!" said Tigger "This game
that we played, helps you to see the
world in a different way."

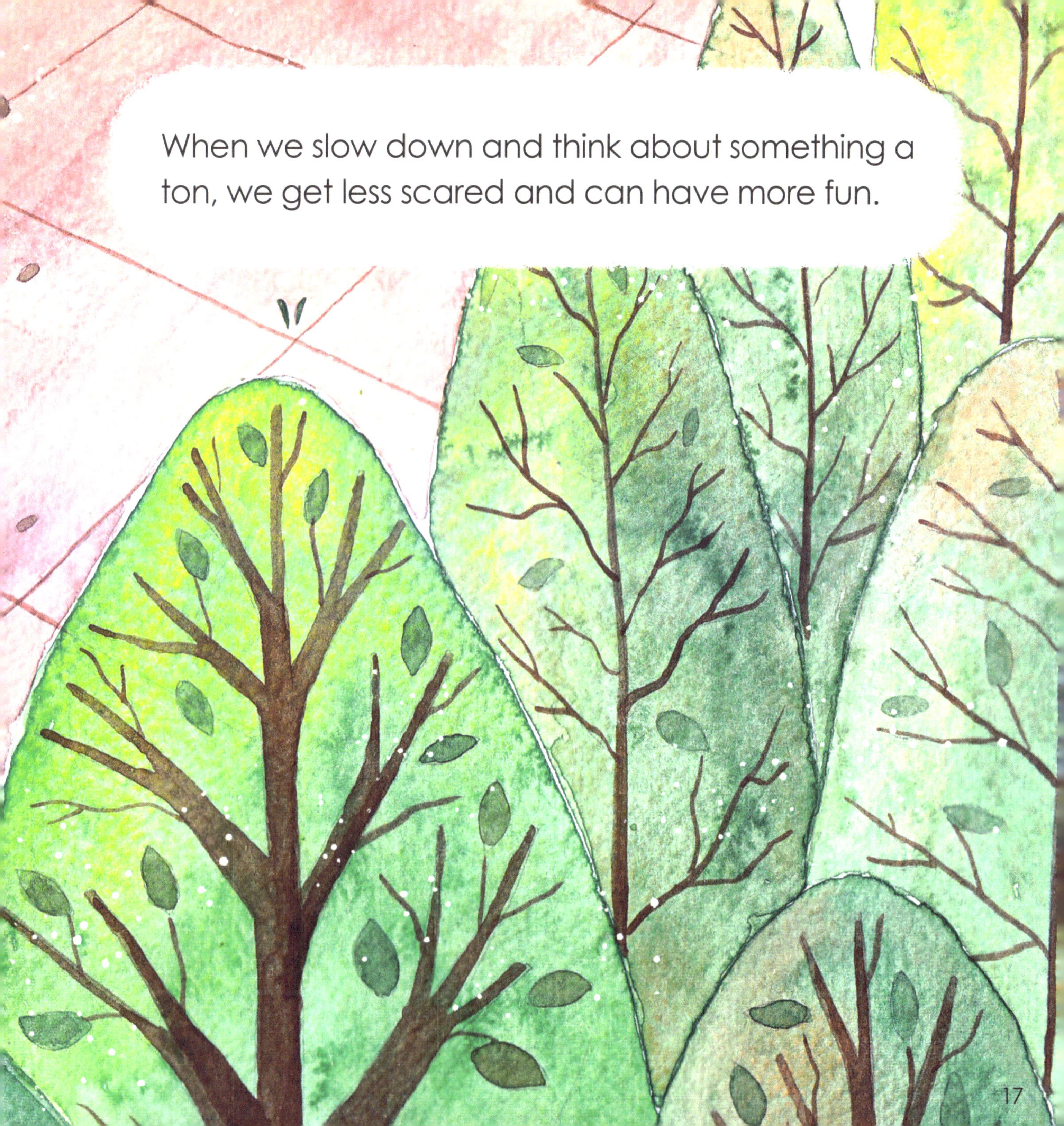

When we slow down and think about something a ton, we get less scared and can have more fun.

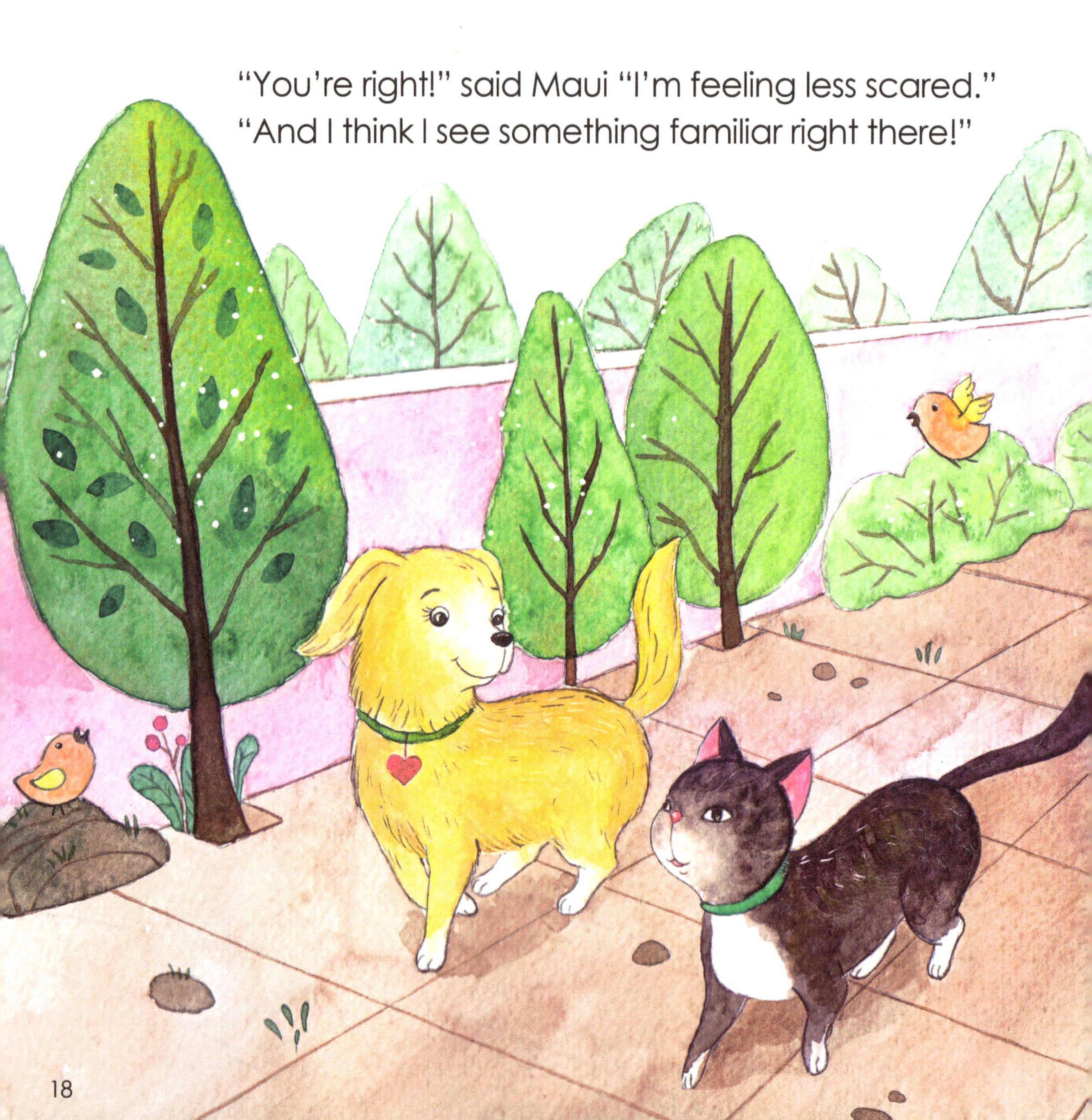

"You're right!" said Maui "I'm feeling less scared."
"And I think I see something familiar right there!"

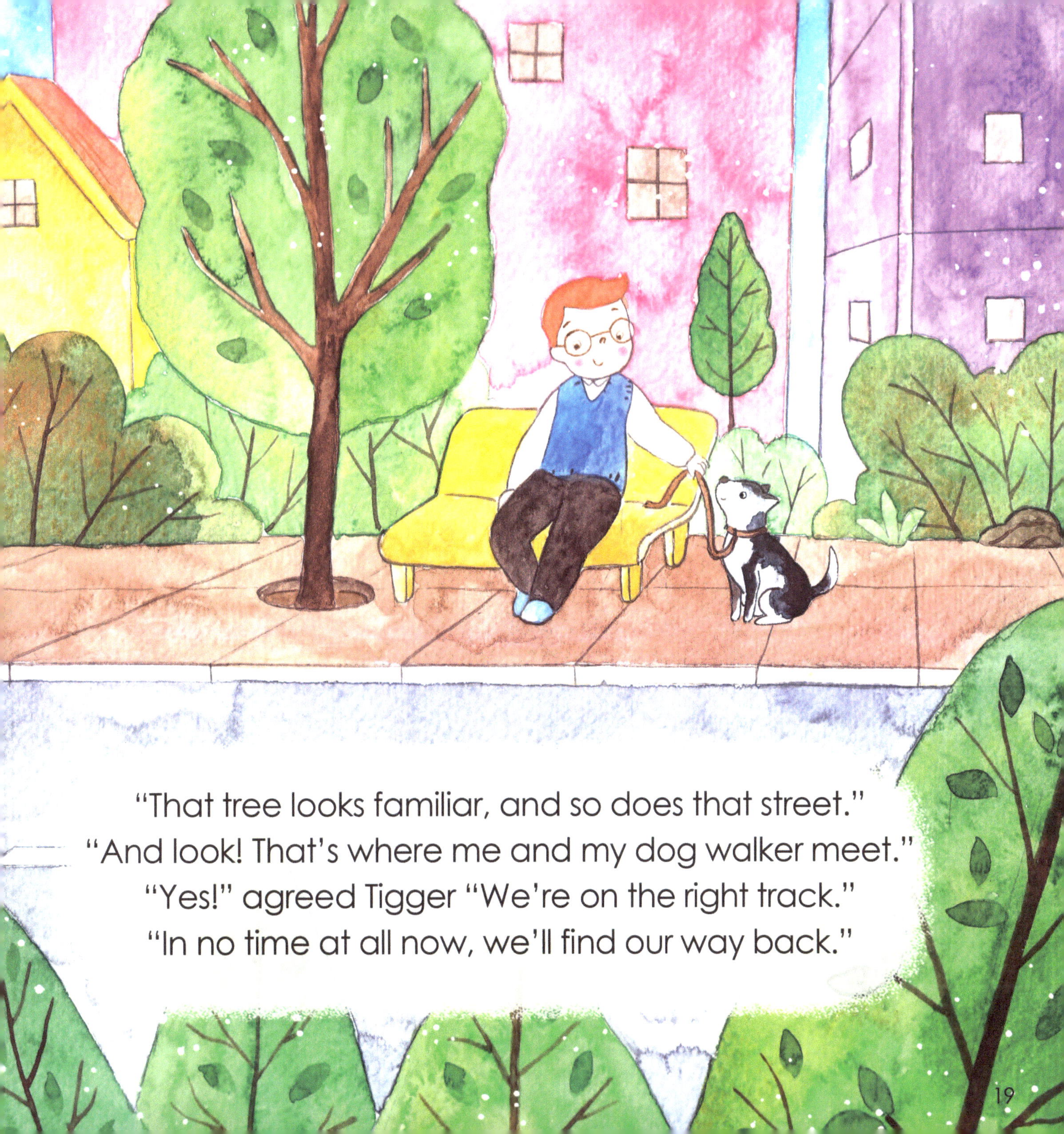

"That tree looks familiar, and so does that street."
"And look! That's where me and my dog walker meet."
"Yes!" agreed Tigger "We're on the right track."
"In no time at all now, we'll find our way back."

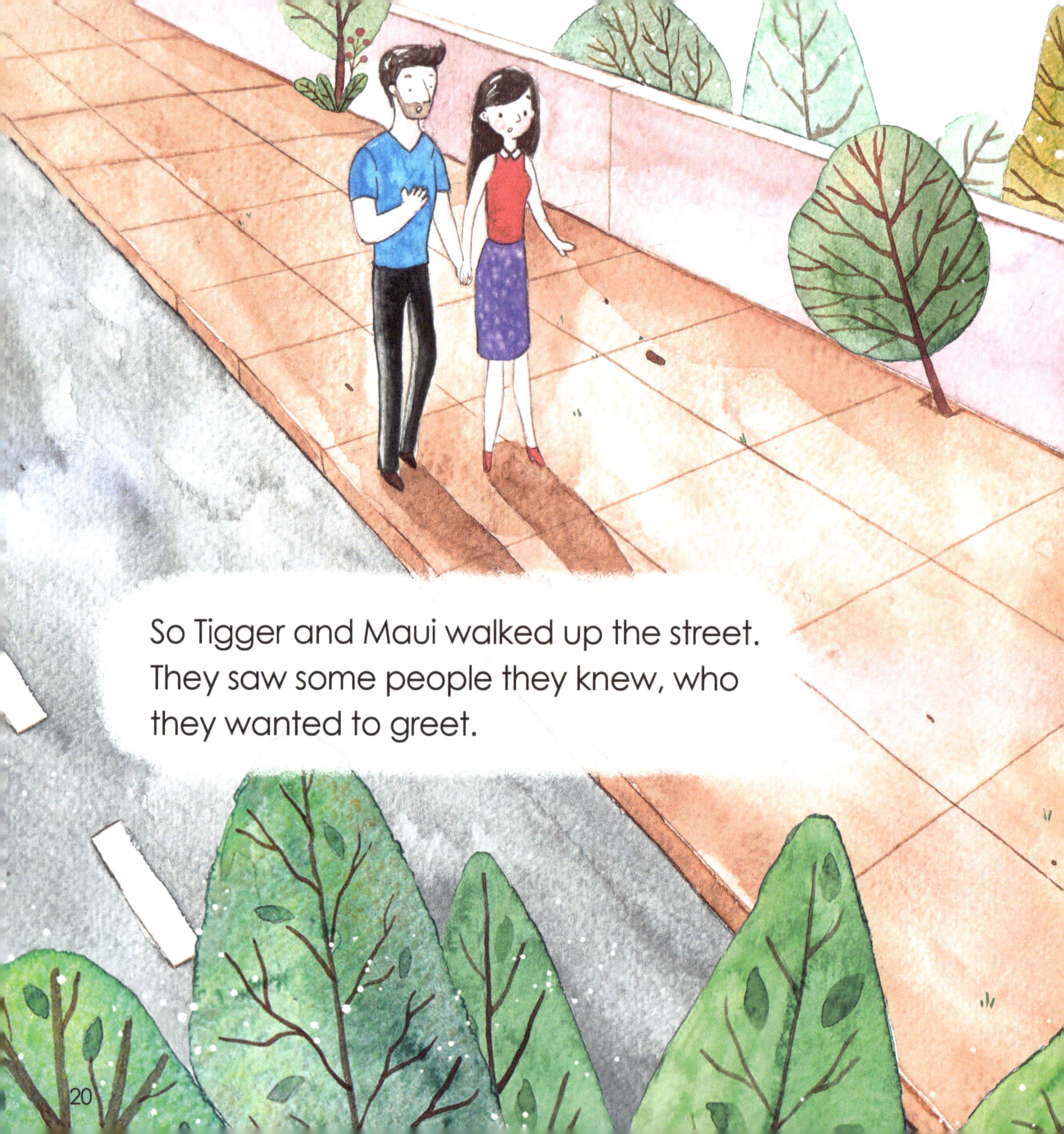

So Tigger and Maui walked up the street.
They saw some people they knew, who
they wanted to greet.

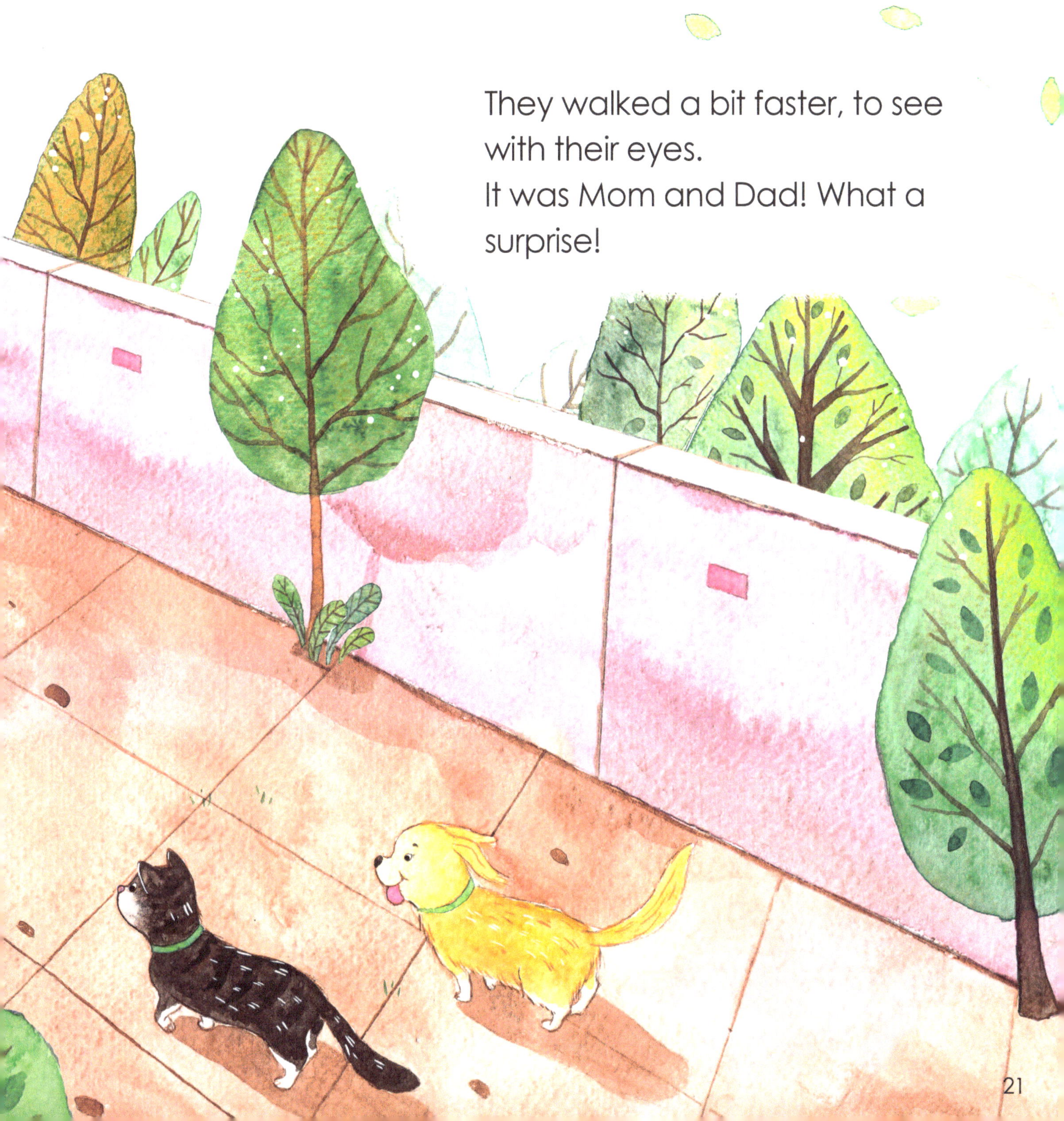

They walked a bit faster, to see with their eyes.
It was Mom and Dad! What a surprise!

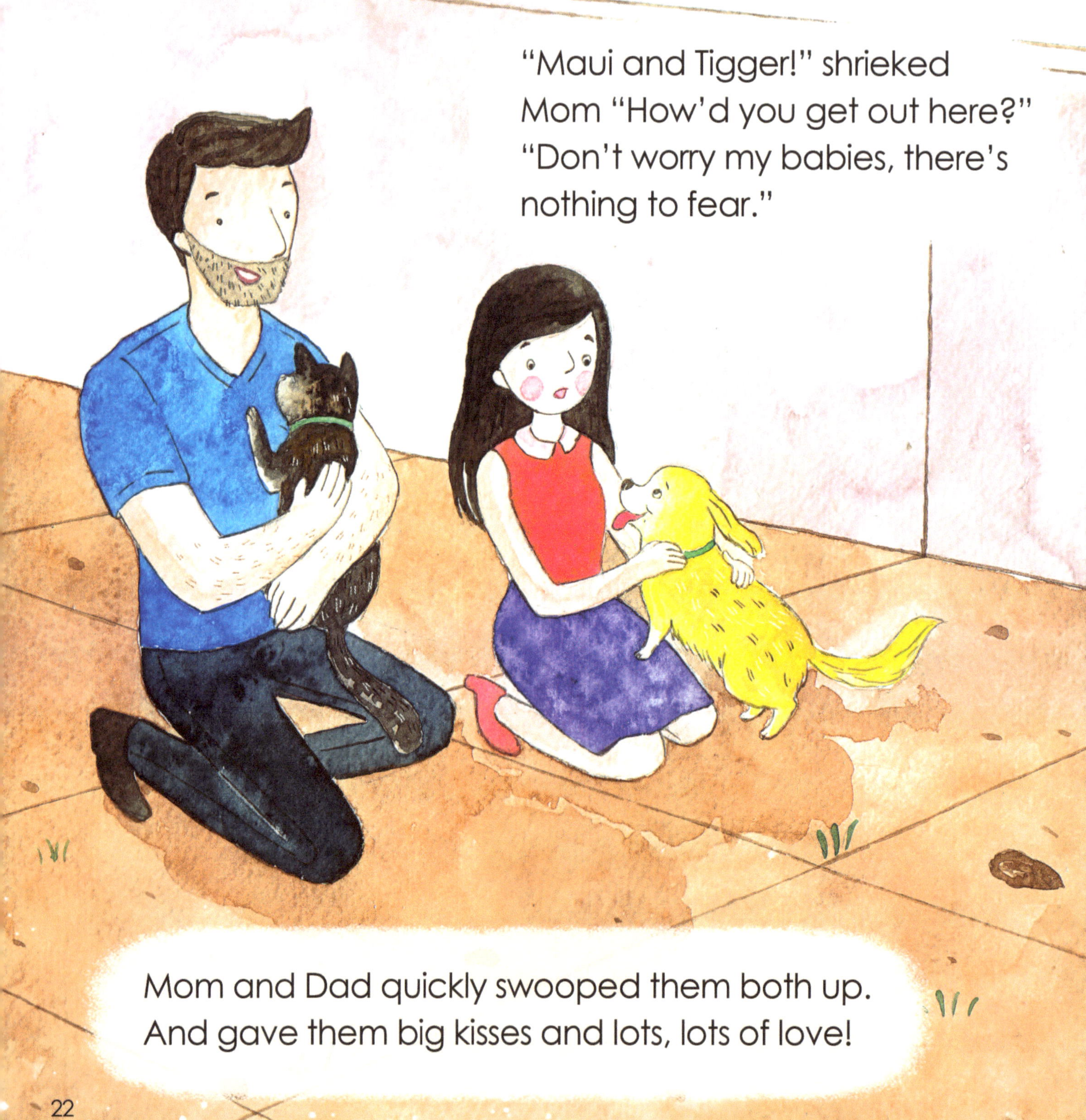

"Maui and Tigger!" shrieked
Mom "How'd you get out here?"
"Don't worry my babies, there's
nothing to fear."

Mom and Dad quickly swooped them both up.
And gave them big kisses and lots, lots of love!

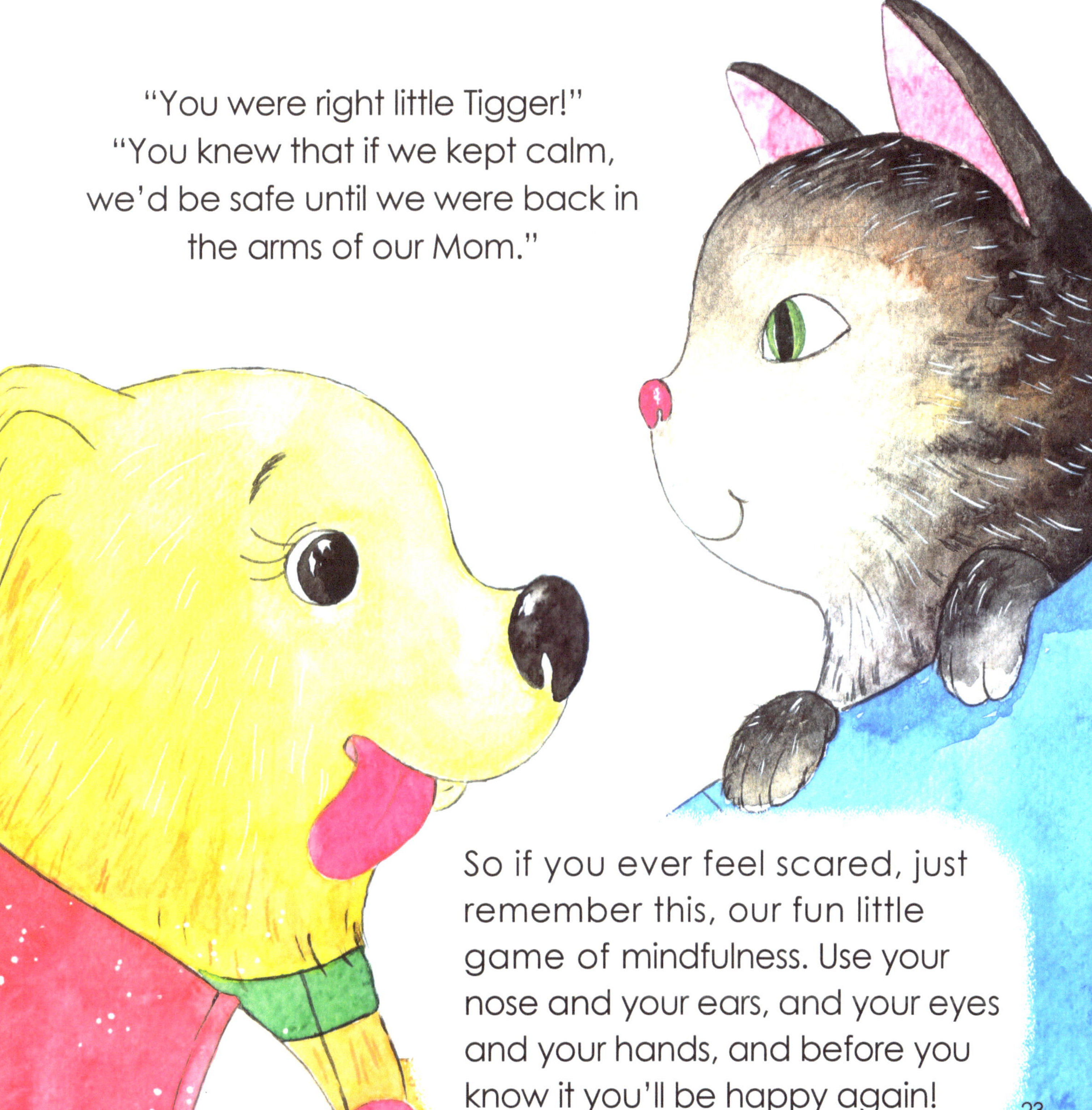

"You were right little Tigger!"
"You knew that if we kept calm,
we'd be safe until we were back in
the arms of our Mom."

So if you ever feel scared, just
remember this, our fun little
game of mindfulness. Use your
nose and your ears, and your eyes
and your hands, and before you
know it you'll be happy again!

23

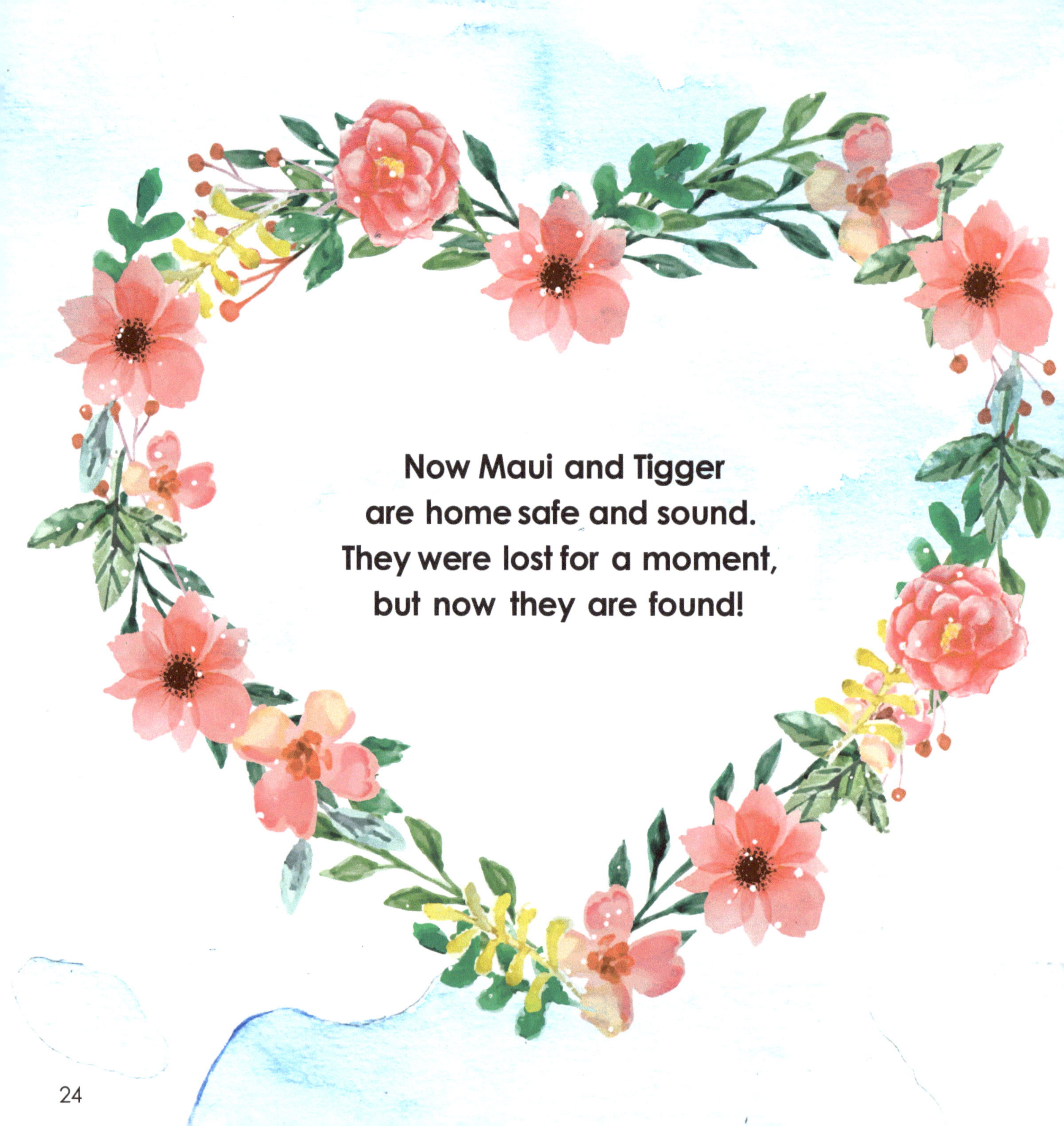

Now Maui and Tigger
are home safe and sound.
They were lost for a moment,
but now they are found!

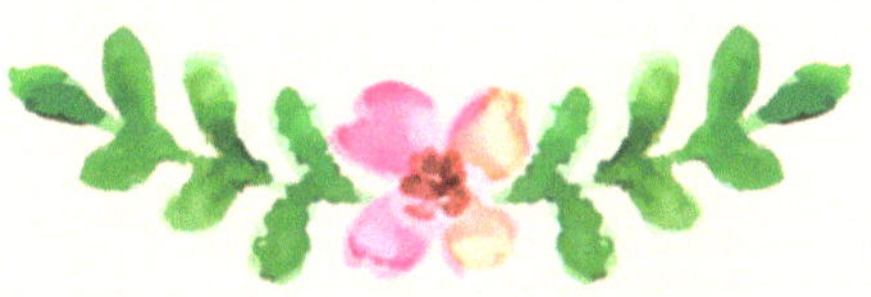

THE END !

www.ingramcontent.com/pod-product-compliance
Lightning Source LLC
Chambersburg PA
CBHW040058240726
48664CB00004B/1237